STEVE HAINES

PAIN IS REALLY STRANGE

ART BY SOPHIE STANDING

SINGING

PUBLISHED BY SINGING DRAGON,
AN IMPRINT OF JESSICA KINGSLEY PUBLISHERS

73 COLLIER STREET
LONDON N1 9BE, UK
AND
400 MARKET STREET,
SUITE 400 PHILADELPHIA,
PA 19106, USA

WWW·SINGINGDRAGON·COM

ISBN 978 1 84819 366 6
EISBN 978 0 85701 212 8

PRINTED AND BOUND IN CHINA·

PAIN IS REALLY STRANGE.

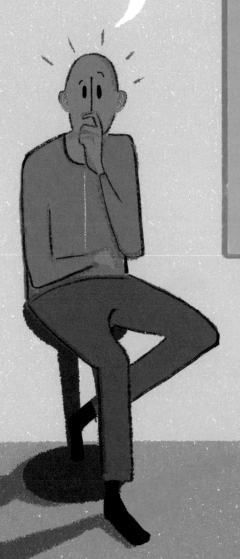

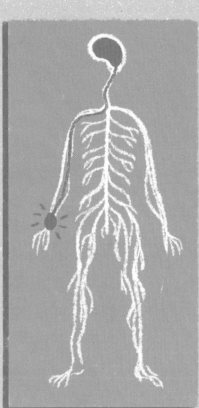

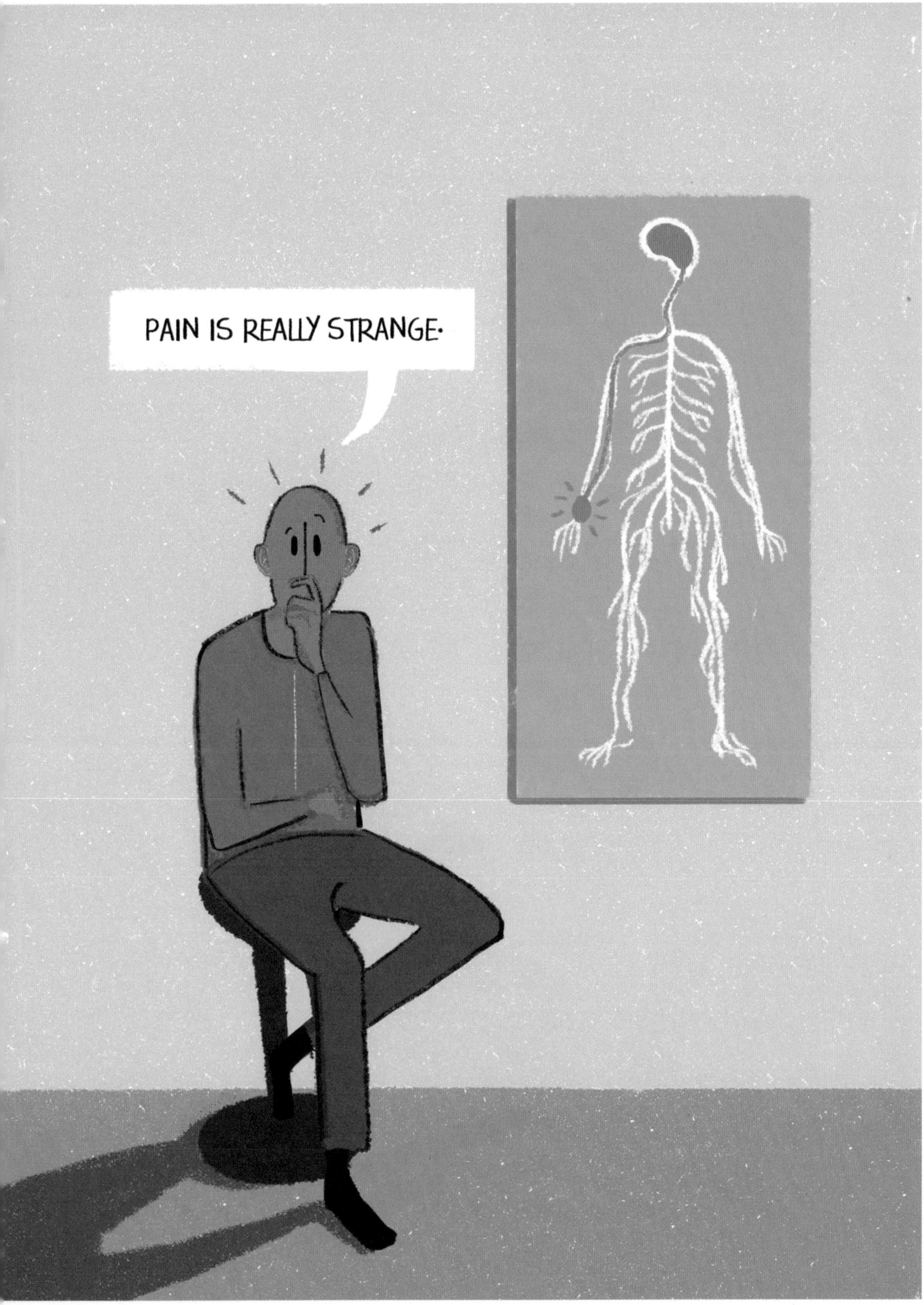

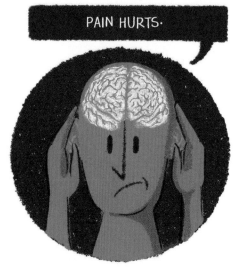

PAIN HURTS.

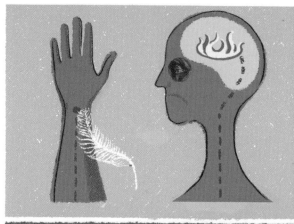

A YOUNG DANCER SPRAINS HER WRIST AND THE PAIN AMPLIFIES UNTIL BEING TOUCHED WITH A FEATHER IS A TERRIFYING BURNING.

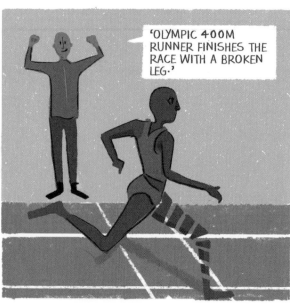

'OLYMPIC 400M RUNNER FINISHES THE RACE WITH A BROKEN LEG.'

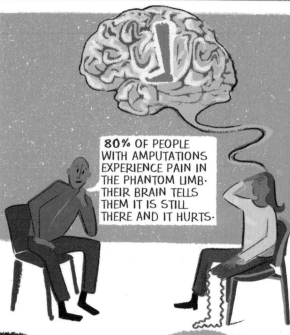

80% OF PEOPLE WITH AMPUTATIONS EXPERIENCE PAIN IN THE PHANTOM LIMB. THEIR BRAIN TELLS THEM IT IS STILL THERE AND IT HURTS.

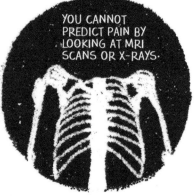

YOU CANNOT PREDICT PAIN BY LOOKING AT MRI SCANS OR X-RAYS.

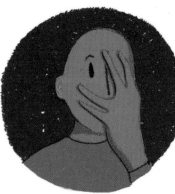

SEEING X-RAYS AND MRI SCANS MAY ACTUALLY MAKE YOU MORE LIKELY TO EXPERIENCE PAIN AS THEY LOOK SCARY.

IN FACT MANY OF US HAVE TORN TISSUES, DISC BULGES AND KNARLY LOOKING BONES WITH NO PAIN.

In the London 2012 Olympics Manteo Mitchell ran the first leg of the heat for the 4x400 metres relay and felt a pop. X-rays revealed afterwards that he broke his left fibula. His team still qualified (Huffington Post 2012).

The dancer's experience is the centre of a great TED talk by Krane (2011). 'Allodynia' is the term for when light touch generates severe pain - the nervous system is confused and sensitized.

IT IS USEFUL TO DIFFERENTIATE CHRONIC PAIN AND ACUTE PAIN. CHRONIC IS USED IF PAIN PERSISTS MORE THAN 3-6 MONTHS.

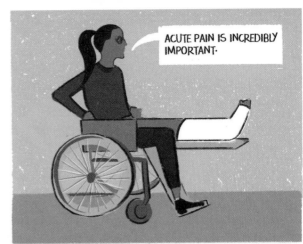

ACUTE PAIN IS INCREDIBLY IMPORTANT.

IT CHANGES HOW WE BEHAVE TO PROTECT TISSUES WHILST THEY REPAIR.

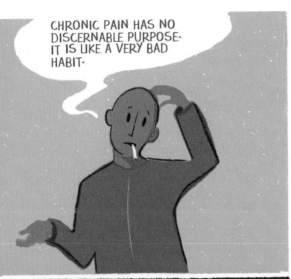

CHRONIC PAIN HAS NO DISCERNABLE PURPOSE. IT IS LIKE A VERY BAD HABIT.

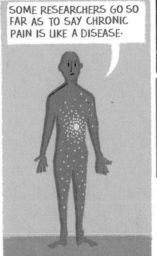

SOME RESEARCHERS GO SO FAR AS TO SAY CHRONIC PAIN IS LIKE A DISEASE.

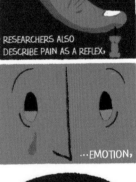

RESEARCHERS ALSO DESCRIBE PAIN AS A REFLEX,

...EMOTION,

...OR MEMORY.

THIS BOOK ATTEMPTS TO LOOK AT HOW PAIN WORKS AND WHAT YOU CAN DO ABOUT IT.

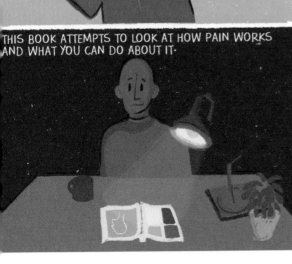

GOOD NEWS: IT TURNS OUT UNDERSTANDING PAIN IS A VERY GOOD WAY OF RELIEVING PAIN.

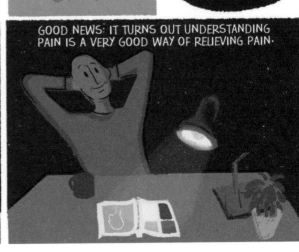

Pain is a disease' (Krane 2011). Pain as 'unresolved emotional trauma held within the body' (Levine and Phillips 2012). '...emerging concepts of maladaptive pain and fear suggest that they share basic neuronal circuits and cellular mechanisms of memory formation' (Sandkühler and Lee 2013).

Reading a big Lancet study on pain education was the inspiration for this book. Michaleff et al (2014) compared interventions for chronic whiplash sufferers. 30 mins of reading on understanding pain and how the nervous system worked, plus 2 phone calls performed as well as 20(!) sessions of physiotherapy. Yowser.

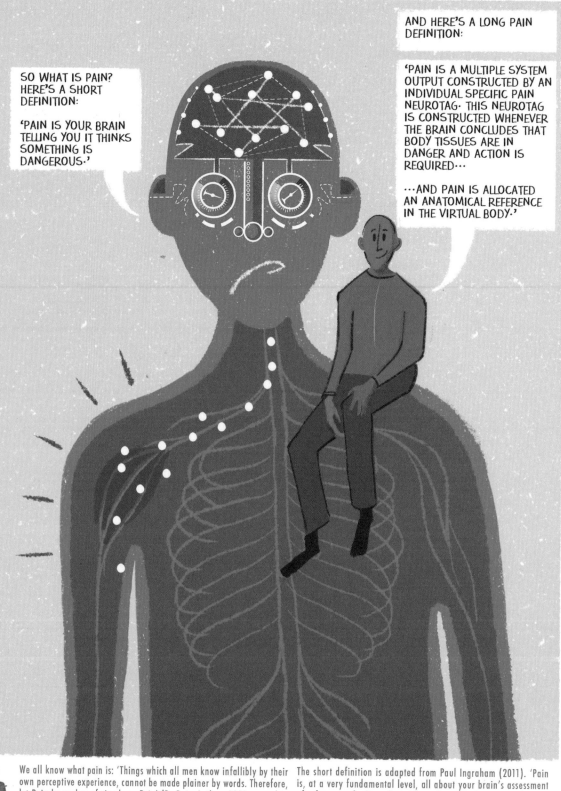

SO WHAT IS PAIN? HERE'S A SHORT DEFINITION:

'PAIN IS YOUR BRAIN TELLING YOU IT THINKS SOMETHING IS DANGEROUS.'

AND HERE'S A LONG PAIN DEFINITION:

'PAIN IS A MULTIPLE SYSTEM OUTPUT CONSTRUCTED BY AN INDIVIDUAL SPECIFIC PAIN NEUROTAG. THIS NEUROTAG IS CONSTRUCTED WHENEVER THE BRAIN CONCLUDES THAT BODY TISSUES ARE IN DANGER AND ACTION IS REQUIRED···

···AND PAIN IS ALLOCATED AN ANATOMICAL REFERENCE IN THE VIRTUAL BODY.'

 We all know what pain is: 'Things which all men know infallibly by their own perceptive experience, cannot be made plainer by words. Therefore, let Pain be spoken of simply as Pain' (Dr Peter Latham 1862, quoted in Bourke 2014a).

The short definition is adapted from Paul Ingraham (2011). 'Pain is, at a very fundamental level, all about your brain's assessment of safety: unsafe things hurt. If your brain thinks you're safe, pain goes down.'

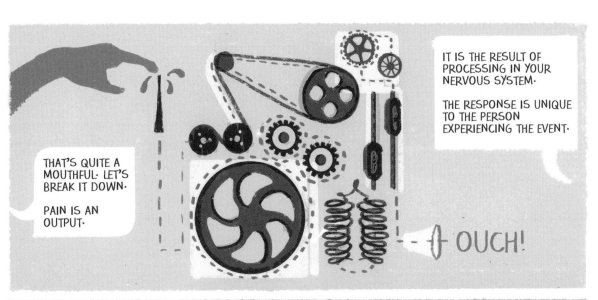

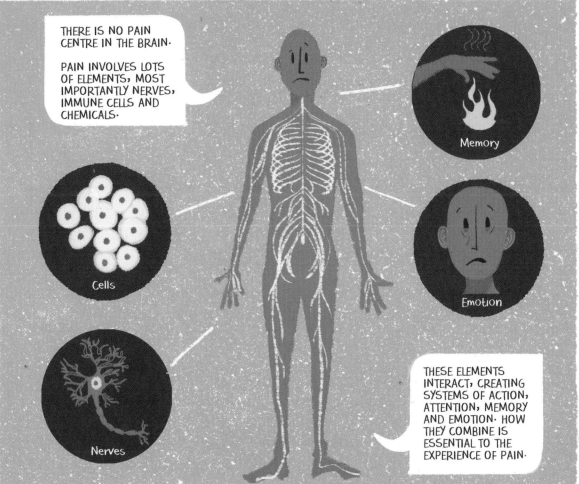

 The long definition is taken from the leading pain researcher Lorimer Moseley (2003). I have changed 'neurosignature' to the shorter 'neurotag'.

Moseley in his talks and writing often states that the brain is evaluating 'How dangerous is this really?' Pain is the answer if the brain decides something is dangerous.

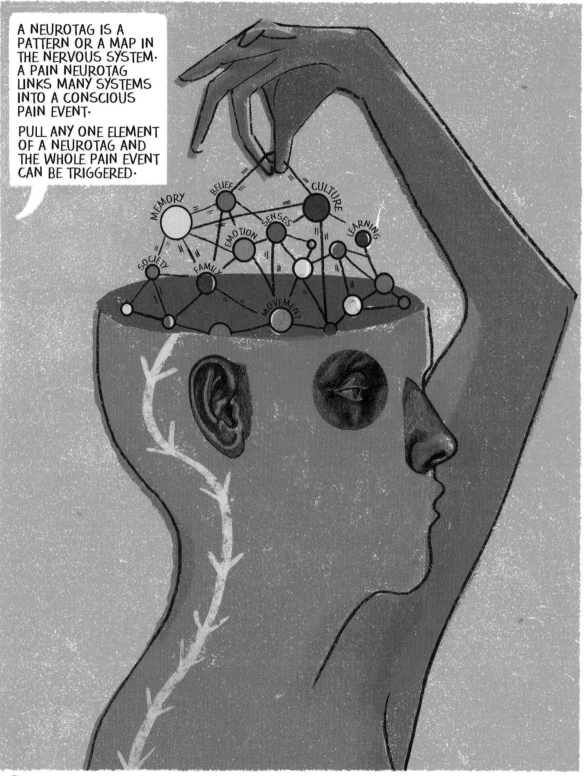

A NEUROTAG IS A PATTERN OR A MAP IN THE NERVOUS SYSTEM. A PAIN NEUROTAG LINKS MANY SYSTEMS INTO A CONSCIOUS PAIN EVENT.

PULL ANY ONE ELEMENT OF A NEUROTAG AND THE WHOLE PAIN EVENT CAN BE TRIGGERED.

 'We can think of pain as a conscious experience that emerges in response to activity in a particular network of brain cells that are spread across the brain. We can call the network a "neurotag" and we can call the brain cells that make up the neurotag "member brain cells"' (Moseley 2012b).

THE NERVOUS SYSTEM RECEIVES DANGER SIGNALS FROM TISSUES AND CELLS THAT ARE DRY, OXYGEN DEPLETED, DAMAGED OR INFLAMED.

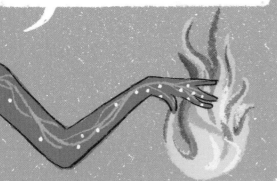

IN ACUTE SITUATIONS, NOCICEPTION, THE FANCY NAME FOR DANGER SIGNALS, USUALLY GENERATES PAIN THAT IS WELL CORRELATED TO DAMAGE. (NOT ALWAYS - REMEMBER THE OLYMPIC RUNNER WITH THE BROKEN LEG.)

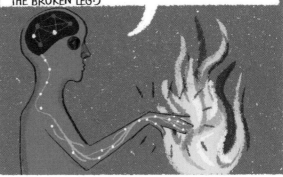

THE BRAIN EVALUATES THE DANGER SIGNALS IN RELATIONSHIP TO EVERYTHING ELSE IT IS PROCESSING.

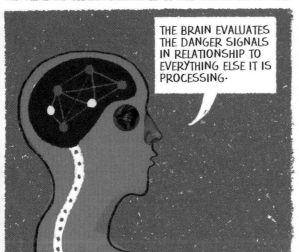

PAIN IS THE MOMENT WHEN YOUR BRAIN DECIDES SOMETHING IS UNSAFE AND YOU NEED TO KNOW ABOUT IT.

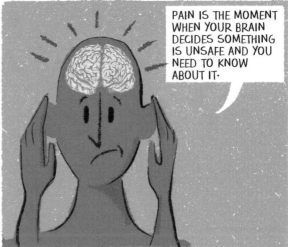

THE BRAIN USES THE BODY TO CREATE A WARNING SIGNAL. THE MIND AND THE BODY ARE INEXORABLY LINKED; THERE IS NO SUCH THING AS PURE THOUGHT. CHANGES IN THE BRAIN ALWAYS RESULT IN A CHANGE IN PHYSIOLOGY SOMEWHERE IN THE BODY.

THE 'VIRTUAL BODY' IS THE NEUROTAG OF THE BODY. IT INCLUDES THE CURRENT MAP OF THE BODY, AND THE HISTORY AND PREDICTION OF HAVING A BODY. WE CAN SAY THE BRAIN USES THE BODY AS A DASHBOARD. PAIN IS A FLASHING RED LIGHT THAT IS HARD TO IGNORE.

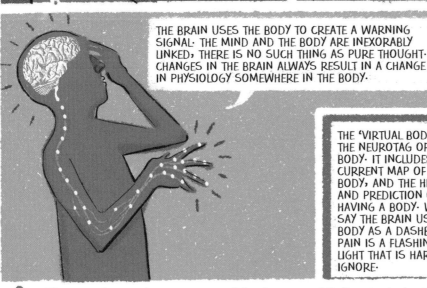

 'The neurons that carry those messages are called nociceptors, or danger receptors. We call the system that detects and transmits noxious events "nociception".

Critically, nociception is neither sufficent nor necessary for pain. But most of the time pain is associated with some nociception' (Moseley 2012b).

YOUR PERCEPTION OF REALITY IS CREATED BY NEURONS. HOW NEURONS INTERACT IS THE BEGINNING AND END OF EVERYTHING. YOUR FEELINGS, MEMORIES AND DREAMS ARE WRITTEN BY THESE CELLS.

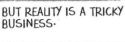
BUT REALITY IS A TRICKY BUSINESS.

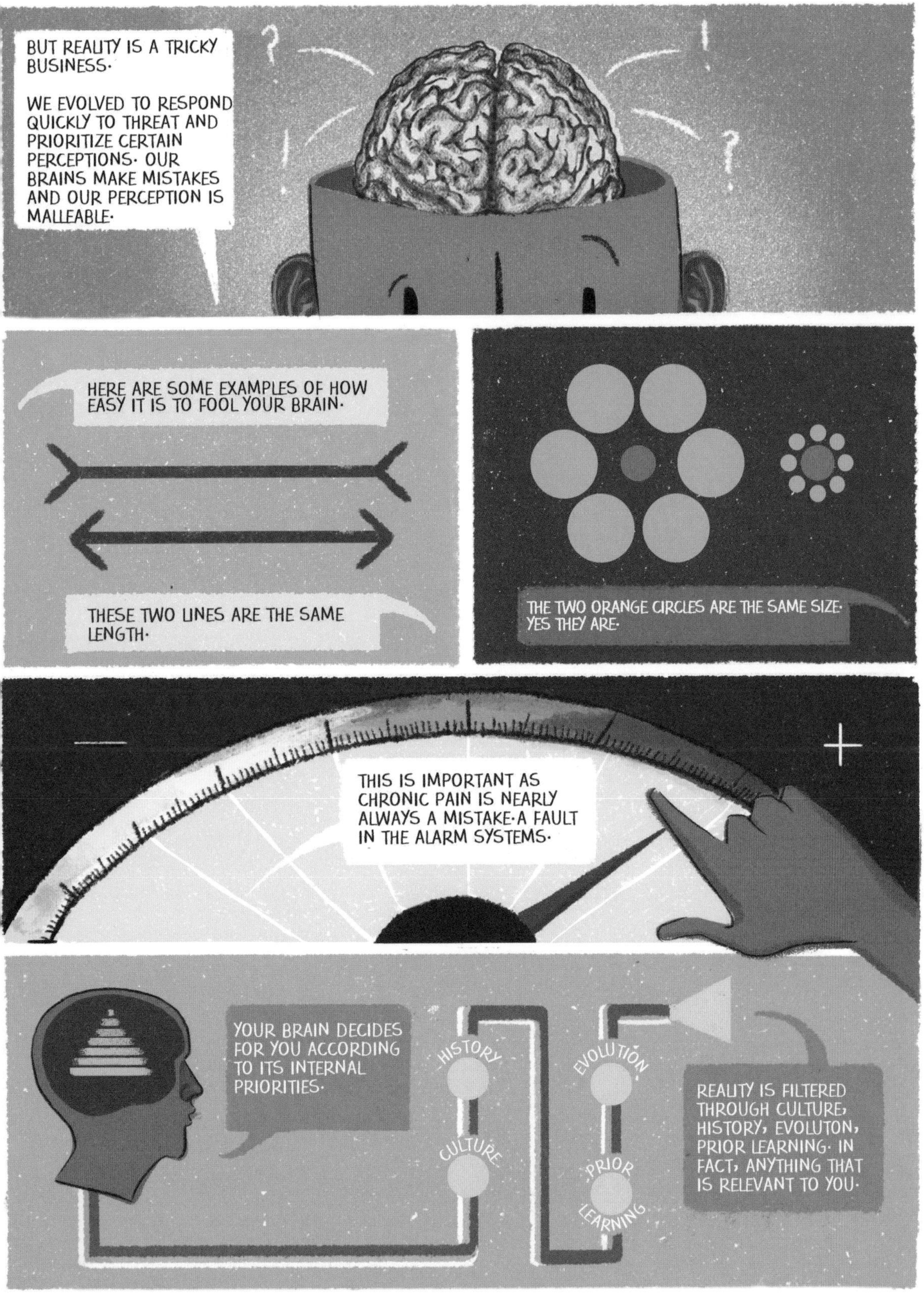

WE EVOLVED TO RESPOND QUICKLY TO THREAT AND PRIORITIZE CERTAIN PERCEPTIONS. OUR BRAINS MAKE MISTAKES AND OUR PERCEPTION IS MALLEABLE.

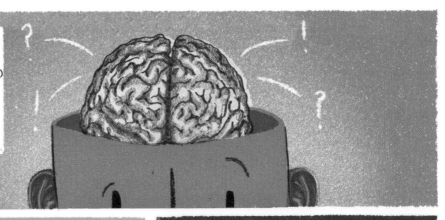

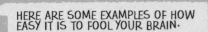
HERE ARE SOME EXAMPLES OF HOW EASY IT IS TO FOOL YOUR BRAIN.

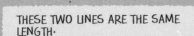
THESE TWO LINES ARE THE SAME LENGTH.

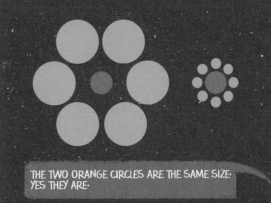
THE TWO ORANGE CIRCLES ARE THE SAME SIZE. YES THEY ARE.

THIS IS IMPORTANT AS CHRONIC PAIN IS NEARLY ALWAYS A MISTAKE. A FAULT IN THE ALARM SYSTEMS.

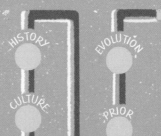

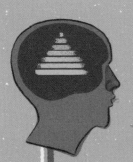
YOUR BRAIN DECIDES FOR YOU ACCORDING TO ITS INTERNAL PRIORITIES.

HISTORY

CULTURE

EVOLUTION

PRIOR LEARNING

REALITY IS FILTERED THROUGH CULTURE, HISTORY, EVOLUTON, PRIOR LEARNING. IN FACT, ANYTHING THAT IS RELEVANT TO YOU.

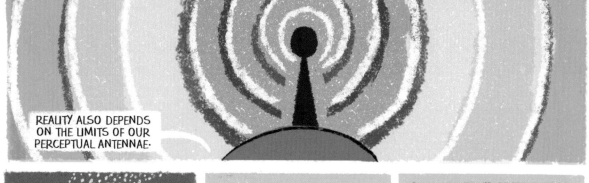

REALITY ALSO DEPENDS ON THE LIMITS OF OUR PERCEPTUAL ANTENNAE.

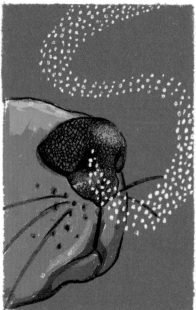

YOU CANNOT SMELL WHAT A DOG SMELLS.

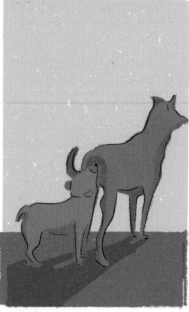

THAT IS OFTEN A GOOD THING.

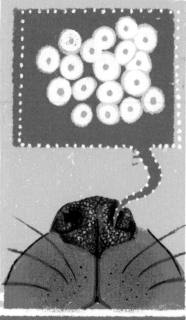

SOME DOGS CAN SMELL CANCER OR EPILEPSY. THAT WOULD BE QUITE USEFUL.

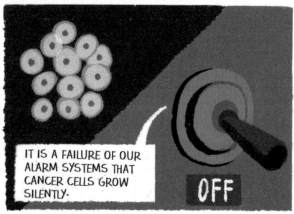

IT IS A FAILURE OF OUR ALARM SYSTEMS THAT CANCER CELLS GROW SILENTLY.

OFF

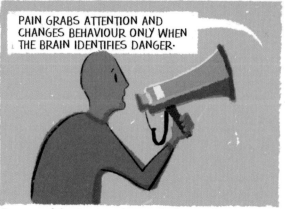

PAIN GRABS ATTENTION AND CHANGES BEHAVIOUR ONLY WHEN THE BRAIN IDENTIFIES DANGER.

Dogs 'sniff out prostate cancer with 98% accuracy' (Medical News Today 2014). 'Reports suggest that some dogs can be trained to anticipate epileptic seizures' (Kirton et al 2008).

Two causes of chronic pain are known to involve more than sensitization: Cancer pain is often intractable and emerges when tumours grow and continuously compress surrounding structures. Neuropathic pain, where the nerve structure is damaged, is also a special case.

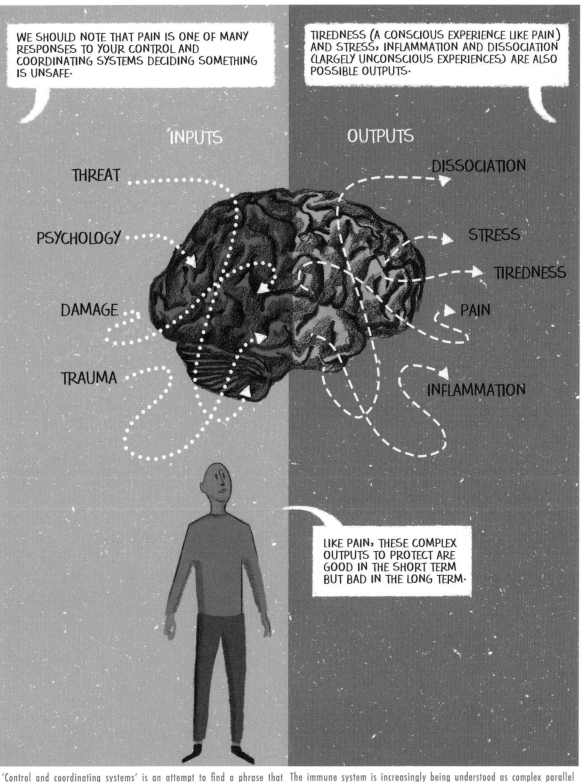

'Control and coordinating systems' is an attempt to find a phrase that honours intelligence as not just about neurons in the brain. Intelligence is an emergent phenomenon generated by trillions of cells communicating throughout the body.

The immune system is increasingly being understood as complex parallel intelligence in the body with memory and learning and a sophisticated range of responses to threat. The immune system is sensitized in chronic inflammation (Thacker et al 2007).

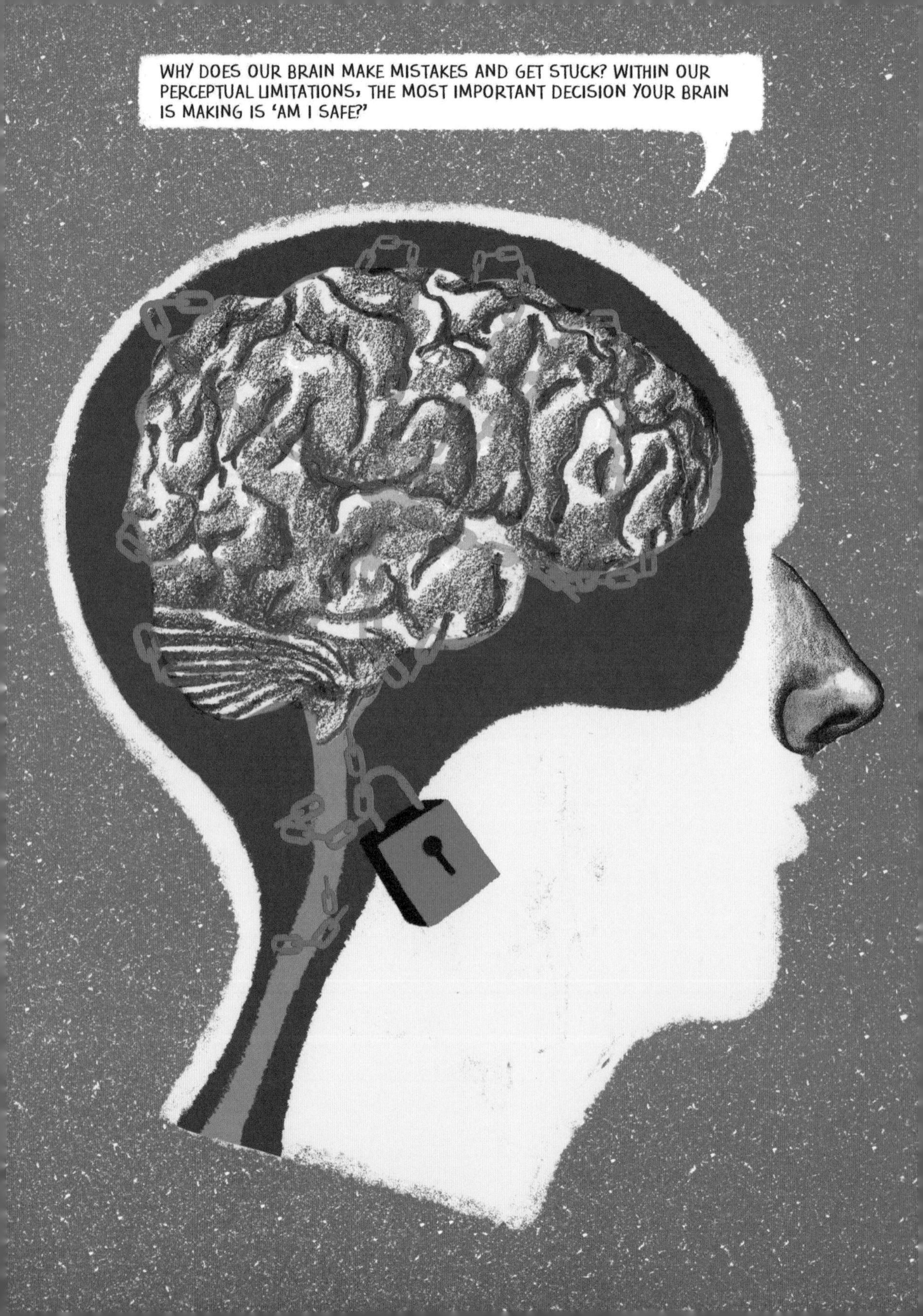
WHY DOES OUR BRAIN MAKE MISTAKES AND GET STUCK? WITHIN OUR PERCEPTUAL LIMITATIONS, THE MOST IMPORTANT DECISION YOUR BRAIN IS MAKING IS 'AM I SAFE?'

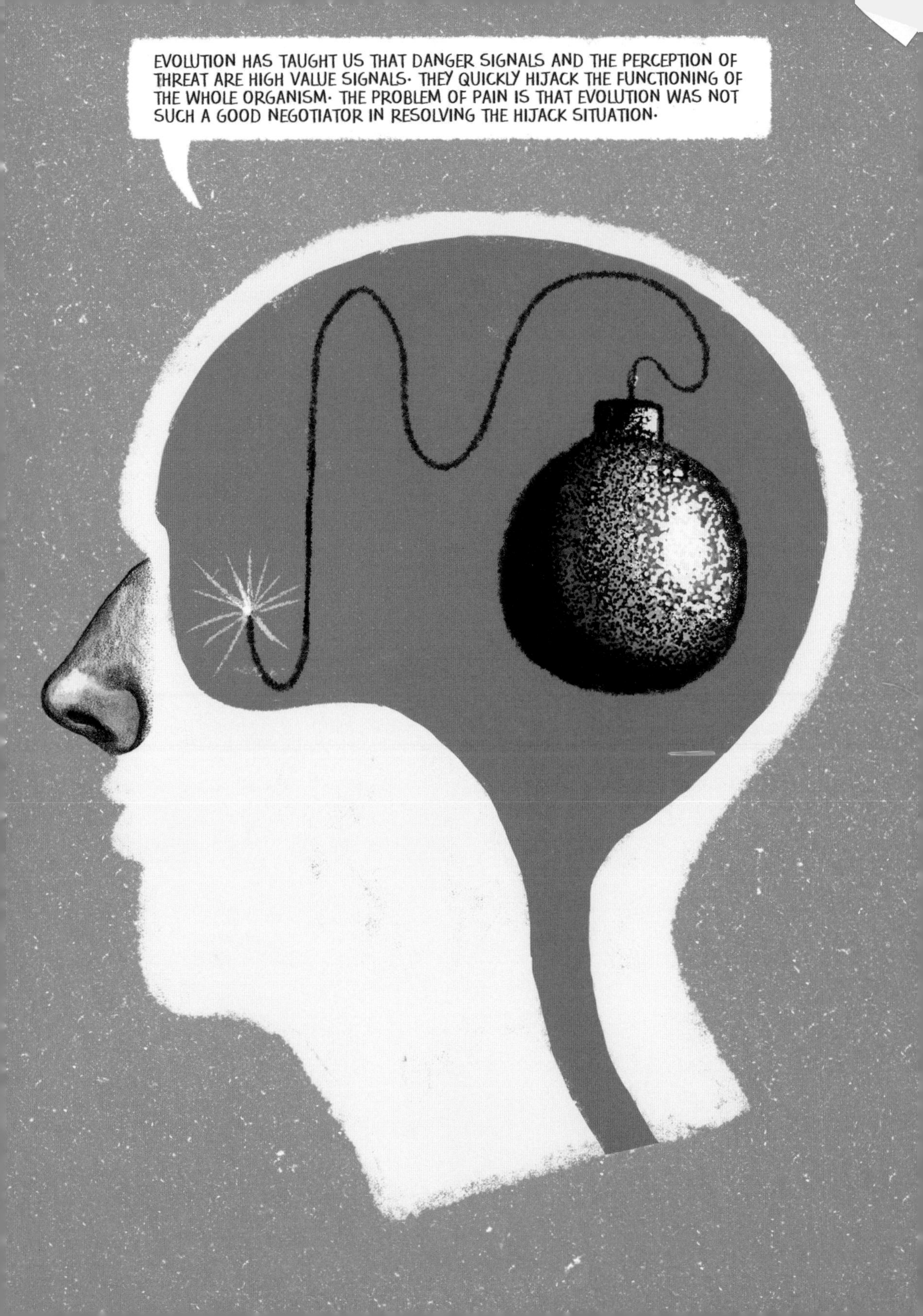
EVOLUTION HAS TAUGHT US THAT DANGER SIGNALS AND THE PERCEPTION OF THREAT ARE HIGH VALUE SIGNALS. THEY QUICKLY HIJACK THE FUNCTIONING OF THE WHOLE ORGANISM. THE PROBLEM OF PAIN IS THAT EVOLUTION WAS NOT SUCH A GOOD NEGOTIATOR IN RESOLVING THE HIJACK SITUATION.

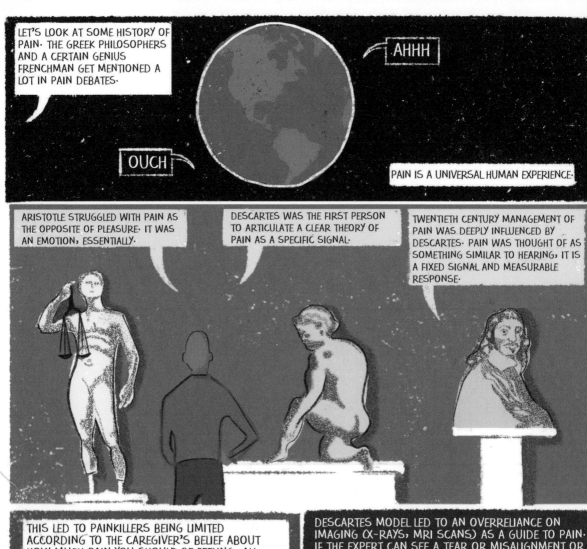

LET'S LOOK AT SOME HISTORY OF PAIN. THE GREEK PHILOSOPHERS AND A CERTAIN GENIUS FRENCHMAN GET MENTIONED A LOT IN PAIN DEBATES.

AHHH

OUCH

PAIN IS A UNIVERSAL HUMAN EXPERIENCE.

ARISTOTLE STRUGGLED WITH PAIN AS THE OPPOSITE OF PLEASURE. IT WAS AN EMOTION, ESSENTIALLY.

DESCARTES WAS THE FIRST PERSON TO ARTICULATE A CLEAR THEORY OF PAIN AS A SPECIFIC SIGNAL.

TWENTIETH CENTURY MANAGEMENT OF PAIN WAS DEEPLY INFLUENCED BY DESCARTES. PAIN WAS THOUGHT OF AS SOMETHING SIMILAR TO HEARING, IT IS A FIXED SIGNAL AND MEASURABLE RESPONSE.

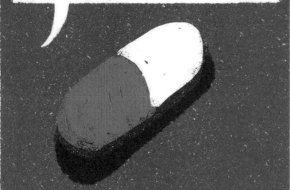

THIS LED TO PAINKILLERS BEING LIMITED ACCORDING TO THE CAREGIVER'S BELIEF ABOUT HOW MUCH PAIN YOU SHOULD BE FEELING. ALL SORTS OF PREJUDICES HAVE BEEN DOCUMENTED. FECKLESS, FOOLISH, FOREIGN, FEMALES LOOK OUT.

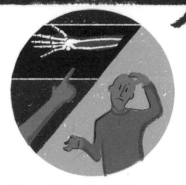

DESCARTES MODEL LED TO AN OVERRELIANCE ON IMAGING (X-RAYS, MRI SCANS) AS A GUIDE TO PAIN. IF THE EXPERT CAN SEE A TEAR OR MISALIGNMENT OR ARTHRITIS THEN THEY WILL TELL YOU THAT CHANGING THE THING THEY CAN SEE WILL REMOVE THE PAIN. THERE IS NOW OVERWHELMING EVIDENCE THIS TYPE OF THINKING IS JUST WRONG.

'The evidence that tissue pathology does not explain chronic pain is overwhelming (e.g., in back pain, neck pain, and knee osteoarthritis)' (Moseley 2012a). It is rare for researchers to use the word 'overwhelming'.

Bourke (2014b) is wonderful on how beliefs have affected treatment. She describes a shocking example of young infants, presumably believed to have limited consciousness and memory, having amputations without anaesthesia as late as the 1970s.

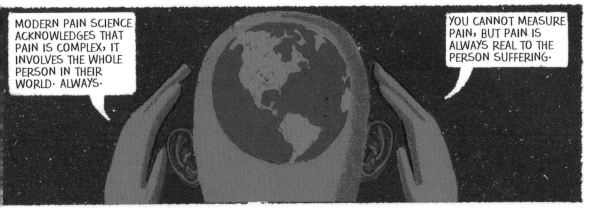

MODERN PAIN SCIENCE ACKNOWLEDGES THAT PAIN IS COMPLEX, IT INVOLVES THE WHOLE PERSON IN THEIR WORLD. ALWAYS.

YOU CANNOT MEASURE PAIN, BUT PAIN IS ALWAYS REAL TO THE PERSON SUFFERING.

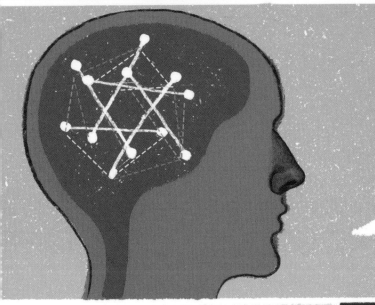

REMEMBER NEUROTAGS ARE PATTERNS IN THE NERVOUS SYSTEM THAT LINK MANY SYSTEMS TOGETHER. THEY ARE THE FOUNDATION OF REALITY AND WHAT WE KNOW.

A PAIN NEUROTAG OVERLAPS WITH AND INTERACTS WITH MANY OTHER NEUROTAGS.

OH DEAR, THAT MEANS LOTS OF THINGS CAN TRIGGER HURT.

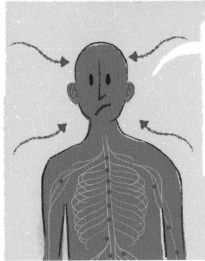

PAIN IS SO MUCH MORE THAN SIGNALS OF DANGER FROM THE TISSUES. IT IS ALSO MUCH MORE THAN BLOCKED EMOTIONS AND BELIEF SYSTEMS. IN FACT THE EXPERIENCE OF PAIN CAN DEPEND ON ANYTHING THAT CAN EFFECT YOU.

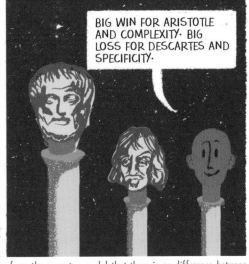

BIG WIN FOR ARISTOTLE AND COMPLEXITY. BIG LOSS FOR DESCARTES AND SPECIFICITY.

'Anyone claiming to be "in pain" is in pain' (Bourke 2014a). Pain is 'elusive'; it is a 'complex experience that can only be measured by the verbal reports of patients' (Cervero 2012).

It follows from the neurotag model that there is no difference between emotional pain and physical pain. Similarly, pain and suffering can be used interchangeably, though pain is described by using the body as a reference and suffering is more often expressed as mental angst.

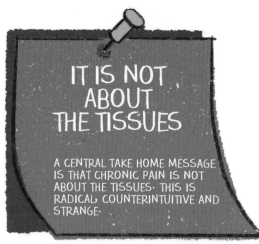

IT IS NOT ABOUT THE TISSUES

A CENTRAL TAKE HOME MESSAGE IS THAT CHRONIC PAIN IS NOT ABOUT THE TISSUES. THIS IS RADICAL, COUNTERINTUITIVE AND STRANGE.

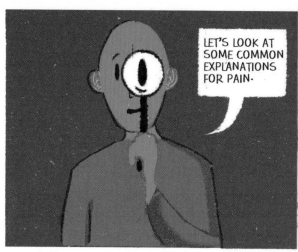

LET'S LOOK AT SOME COMMON EXPLANATIONS FOR PAIN.

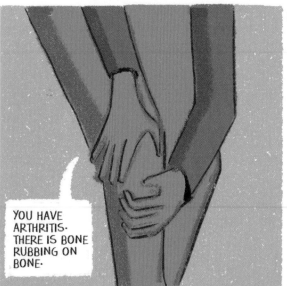

YOU HAVE ARTHRITIS. THERE IS BONE RUBBING ON BONE.

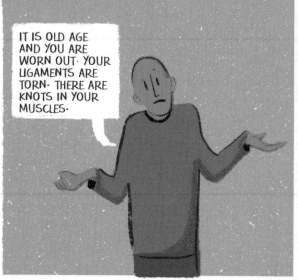

IT IS OLD AGE AND YOU ARE WORN OUT. YOUR LIGAMENTS ARE TORN. THERE ARE KNOTS IN YOUR MUSCLES.

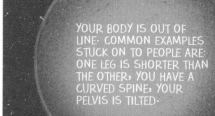

YOUR BODY IS OUT OF LINE. COMMON EXAMPLES STUCK ON TO PEOPLE ARE: ONE LEG IS SHORTER THAN THE OTHER, YOU HAVE A CURVED SPINE, YOUR PELVIS IS TILTED.

 Getting old is not associated with an increase in back pain. In a large study 'there were no meaningful differences in the frequency of low back pain between younger and older individuals' (Lederman 2010).

Alignment does not predict back pain. Excessive spinal curves 'failed to show an association with back pain' (Lederman 2010). 'Modern scientific evidence clearly shows that the importance of most bio-"mechanical" problems has been greatly exaggerated' (Ingraham 2014).

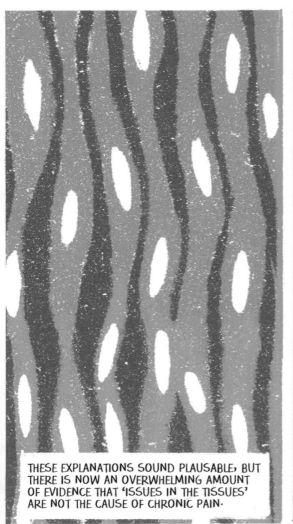

THESE EXPLANATIONS SOUND PLAUSABLE, BUT THERE IS NOW AN OVERWHELMING AMOUNT OF EVIDENCE THAT 'ISSUES IN THE TISSUES' ARE NOT THE CAUSE OF CHRONIC PAIN.

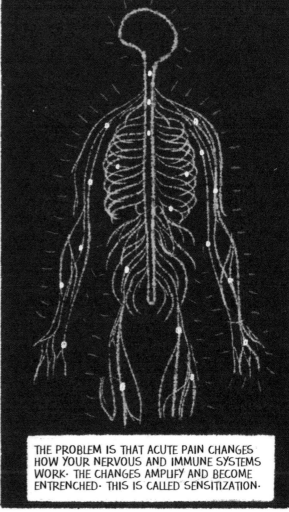

THE PROBLEM IS THAT ACUTE PAIN CHANGES HOW YOUR NERVOUS AND IMMUNE SYSTEMS WORK. THE CHANGES AMPLIFY AND BECOME ENTRENCHED. THIS IS CALLED SENSITIZATION.

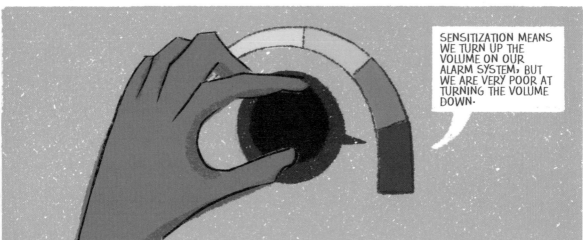

SENSITIZATION MEANS WE TURN UP THE VOLUME ON OUR ALARM SYSTEM, BUT WE ARE VERY POOR AT TURNING THE VOLUME DOWN.

'Joint pains are often described as grinding.' This word is a 'brain derived construction' used because it 'makes sense mechanically'. 'We all have worn out joint surfaces and little bony outgrowths,' '...but most people with worn joints will never know about it' (Butler and Moseley 2003).

Shoulder surgeons, examining the relationship between the severity of rotator cuff (a group of muscles and ligaments in the shoulder) disease and pain, found 'symptoms of pain do not correlate with rotator cuff tear severity' (Dunn et al 2014). Wow, seeing a tear is often used to justify surgery.

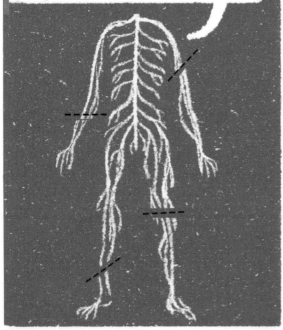

ONE CLEAR PIECE OF EVIDENCE THAT SENSITIZATION IS THE PROBLEM IS THAT AT VARIOUS STAGES DOCTORS HAVE TRIED TO CUT THE NERVES FROM CHRONICALLY PAINFUL BODY AREAS TO STOP THE PAIN.

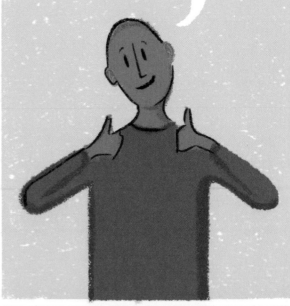

THE REASONING WAS THAT IF YOU STOP THE SIGNAL FROM THE TISSUES YOU WILL NO LONGER FEEL PAIN.

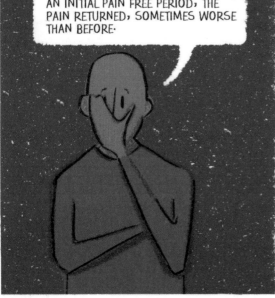

INTENSE ABDOMINAL PAIN IN CANCER PATIENTS WAS TREATED BY CUTTING NERVES IN THE SPINAL CORD. AFTER AN INITIAL PAIN FREE PERIOD, THE PAIN RETURNED, SOMETIMES WORSE THAN BEFORE.

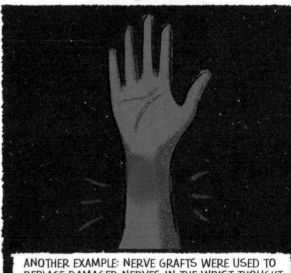

ANOTHER EXAMPLE: NERVE GRAFTS WERE USED TO REPLACE DAMAGED NERVES IN THE WRIST THOUGHT TO BE CAUSING 'DESPERATE BURNING AND TENDERNESS'. WHEN THE GRAFTS HEALED AND NEW HEALTHY TISSUE WAS IN PLACE EVERY PATIENT EXPERIENCED EXACTLY THE SAME HAND PAIN AS BEFORE.

Cervero (2012) describes surgeons in the 1950s cutting bits of the spinal cord to stop severe pain. Initially, on terminal cancer patients, the results were spectacularly good. Patients who lived longer began, tragically, to get pain sensations equal to or worse than the original experience.

Wall (2000) describes wrist surgery to repair median nerves. The patients had improved hand control but, Wall states, 'angry nerve cells' in the cord had become hyperexcitable and were the cause of the ongoing pain.

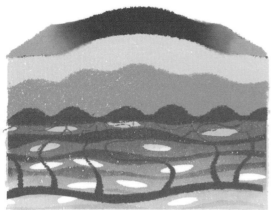

ANOTHER CLEAR PIECE OF EVIDENCE AGAINST TISSUE BEING THE CAUSE OF PAIN IS THAT TISSUE HEALING COMPLETES WITHIN 3-6 MONTHS.

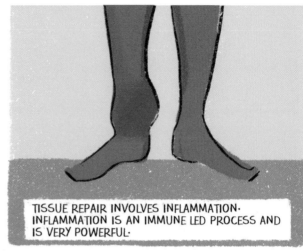

TISSUE REPAIR INVOLVES INFLAMMATION. INFLAMMATION IS AN IMMUNE LED PROCESS AND IS VERY POWERFUL.

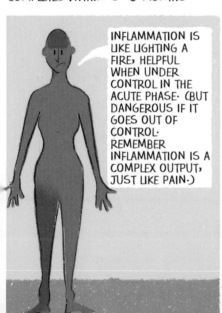

INFLAMMATION IS LIKE LIGHTING A FIRE, HELPFUL WHEN UNDER CONTROL IN THE ACUTE PHASE. (BUT DANGEROUS IF IT GOES OUT OF CONTROL. REMEMBER INFLAMMATION IS A COMPLEX OUTPUT, JUST LIKE PAIN.)

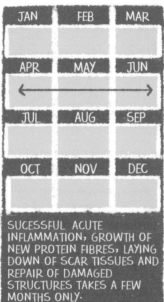

JAN	FEB	MAR
APR	MAY	JUN
JUL	AUG	SEP
OCT	NOV	DEC

SUCCESSFUL ACUTE INFLAMMATION, GROWTH OF NEW PROTEIN FIBRES, LAYING DOWN OF SCAR TISSUES AND REPAIR OF DAMAGED STRUCTURES TAKES A FEW MONTHS ONLY.

AFTER TISSUE HEALING IS COMPLETE THERE MAY BE SOME LOSS OF FUNCTION. YOU MAY NEED TO LEARN TO MOVE DIFFERENTLY, BUT THERE IS NO NEED FOR PAIN.

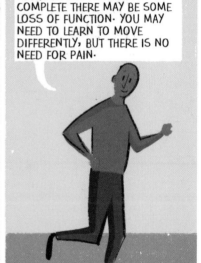

PERSISTENT PAIN, BEYOND THE PERIOD FOR OPTIMUM TISSUE HEALING, MEANS THE BRAIN HAS FORGOTTEN TO TURN OFF THE ALARM SYSTEM. OOPS.

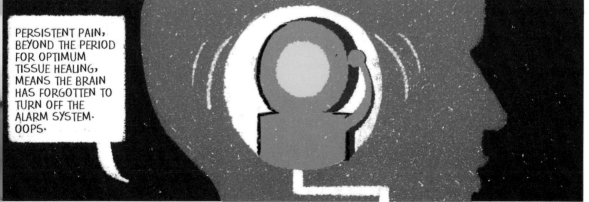

'We know most tissues in the human body heal between 3 - 6 months. It is now well established that ongoing pain is more due to a sensitive nervous system. In other words, the body's alarm system stays in alarm mode after tissues have healed' (Louw 2013).

Medicine 'assumes that injury and pain are the same issue; therefore, an increase in pain means increased tissue injury and increased tissue issues lead to more pain. This model (called the Cartesian model of pain) is over 350 years old, and it's incorrect' (Louw 2014).

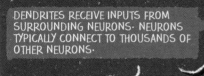

DENDRITES RECEIVE INPUTS FROM SURROUNDING NEURONS. NEURONS TYPICALLY CONNECT TO THOUSANDS OF OTHER NEURONS.

THE CELL BODY COLLECTS ALL THE SIGNALS FROM THE DENDRITES AND COMBINES THE INPUTS INTO A FINAL SIGNAL.

MEMBRANE RECEPTORS TASTE THE SURROUNDING ENVIRONMENT AND CHANGE THE SENSITIVITY OF THE NERVE.

THE AXON EXITS THE CELL BODY AND QUICKLY TRANSMITS THE NERVE IMPULSE.

THE TERMINAL BRANCHES OF AXONS GROW NEW CONNECTIONS TO MORE DENDRITES IF THEY ARE HIGHLY STIMULATED 'CELLS THAT FIRE TOGETHER WIRE TOGETHER.'

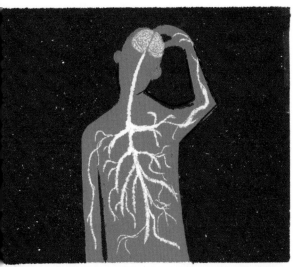

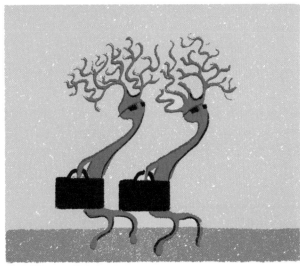

NERVES ARE MUCH MORE COMPLEX THAN YOU PROBABLY REALIZE· A SIMPLE ELECTRIC CABLE OR SIMPLE SWITCH IS AN OVERSIMPLIFICATION·

NERVE CELLS ARE LITTLE AGENTS WITH THEIR OWN AGENDA· THEY ADAPT TO THE DEMANDS PLACED ON THEM·

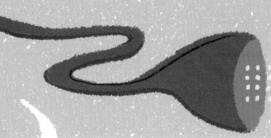

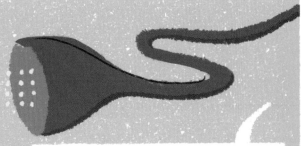

NEURONS CONNECT VIA SYNAPSES· AT THE SYNAPSE, A WAVE OF ELECTRIC CHARGE ALONG THE AXON CAUSES CHEMICALS CALLED NEUROTRANSMITTERS TO BE RELEASED·

ON THE OTHER IDE OF THE SYNAPSE ANOTHER CELL (USUALLY ANOTHER NEURON) ABSORBS THE NEUROTRANSMITTERS VIA MEMBRANE RECEPTORS·

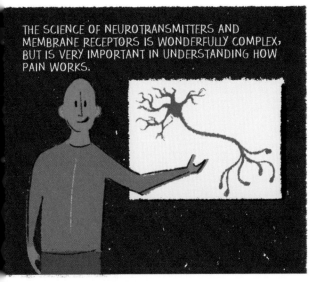

THE SCIENCE OF NEUROTRANSMITTERS AND MEMBRANE RECEPTORS IS WONDERFULLY COMPLEX, BUT IS VERY IMPORTANT IN UNDERSTANDING HOW PAIN WORKS.

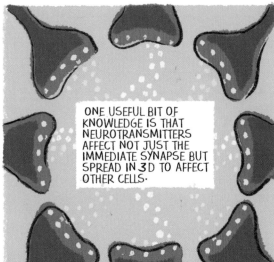

ONE USEFUL BIT OF KNOWLEDGE IS THAT NEUROTRANSMITTERS AFFECT NOT JUST THE IMMEDIATE SYNAPSE BUT SPREAD IN 3D TO AFFECT OTHER CELLS·

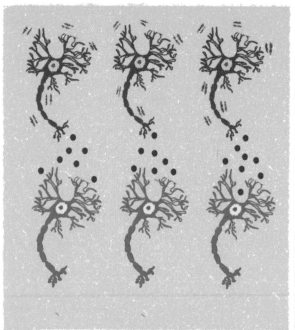

DANGER SIGNALS ARE BAD NEWS THAT TRAVELS FAST. THE ASSOCIATED NEUROTRANSMITTERS QUICKLY AFFECT OTHER CELLS. ANGRY NEURONS SHOUT A LOT.

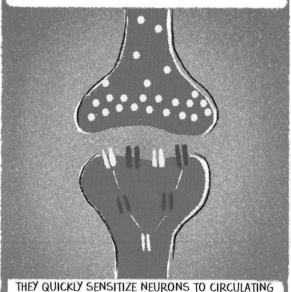

ANOTHER USEFUL BIT OF INFORMATION IS THAT MEMBRANE RECEPTORS CHANGE ALL THE TIME. NEW RECEPTORS ARE INSERTED INTO THE CELL WALL.

THEY QUICKLY SENSITIZE NEURONS TO CIRCULATING STRESS HORMONES, INFLAMMATORY SIGNALS AND DANGER NEUROTRANSMITTERS.

MEMBRANE RECEPTOR CHANGES ARE THE START OF MEMORY AND NEUROPLASTICITY. THE NEW FIELD OF NEUROPLASTICITY HAS DEFINITIVELY PROVED THAT THE CONNECTIONS BETWEEN NEURONS CHANGE ACCORDING TO THE STIMULUS.

Membrane receptors and the activity in synapses are often the targets of pain killing drugs. Anaesthetics have transformed surgery. Common pain killers are very useful drugs.

It is good to regularly review the use of stronger pain killers. Opiates can have difficult side effects, generate addiction, sensitize the nervous system, and tolerance means you will need more. Check YouTube: 'Brainman stops his opiod'.

MEMORY IS REINFORCED BY SPROUTING NEW SYNAPSES AND GREATER INSULATION OF THE NERVE AXONS IN RESPONSE TO REPEATED STIMULATION. THE NERVOUS SYSTEM LEARNS BY CHANGING ITS WIRING.

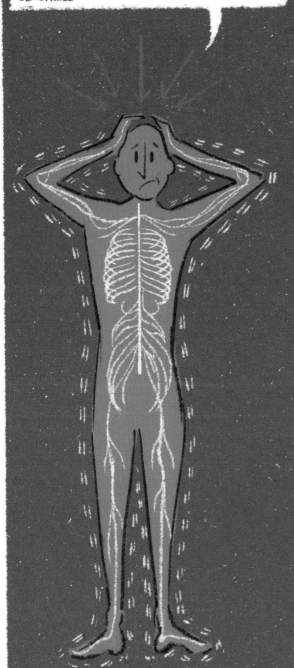

IF WE HAVE LOTS OF DANGER SIGNALS WE LEARN TO AMPLIFY DANGER. OUR NERVOUS SYSTEM BECOMES SENSITIZED.

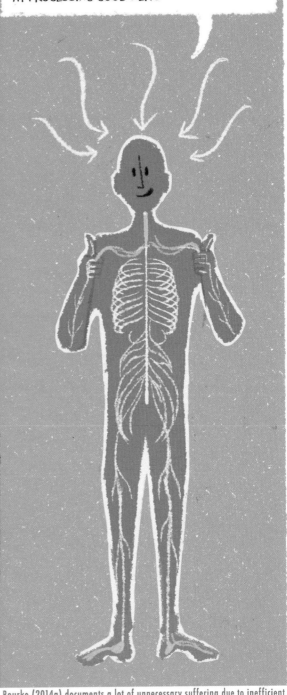

IF WE HAVE LOTS OF GOOD NEWS WE GET BETTER AT PROCESSING GOOD NEWS.

Cervelo (2012) states that end of life pain can cheaply and easily be relieved with improved availability of existing drugs; world wide lack of access to effective pain relief is a political problem leading to needless suffering.

Bourke (2014a) documents a lot of unnecessary suffering due to inefficient administration of stronger prescription pain killers.

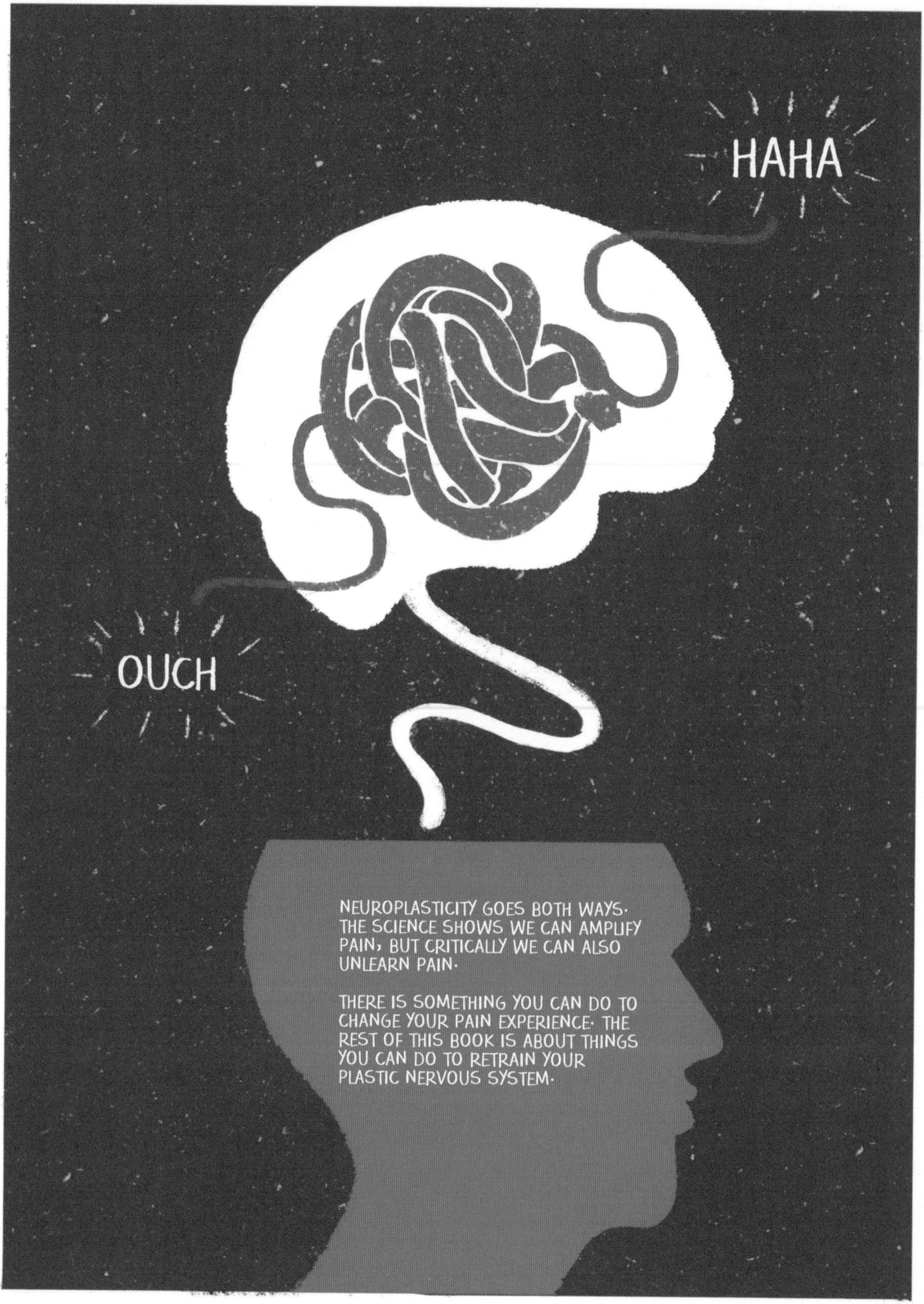
HAHA
OUCH
NEUROPLASTICITY GOES BOTH WAYS. THE SCIENCE SHOWS WE CAN AMPLIFY PAIN, BUT CRITICALLY WE CAN ALSO UNLEARN PAIN.
THERE IS SOMETHING YOU CAN DO TO CHANGE YOUR PAIN EXPERIENCE. THE REST OF THIS BOOK IS ABOUT THINGS YOU CAN DO TO RETRAIN YOUR PLASTIC NERVOUS SYSTEM.

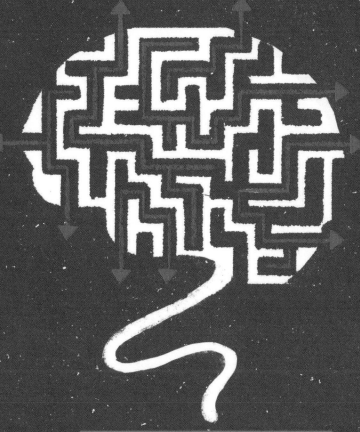

BE CREATIVE.

YOU ARE UNIQUE AND NEED TO
EXPERIMENT TO FIND OUT WHAT WORKS
FOR YOU. THERE IS NO ONE ANSWER
THAT FITS EVERYONE.

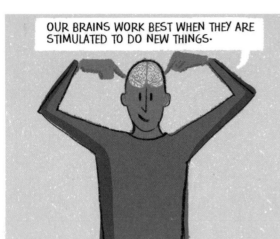

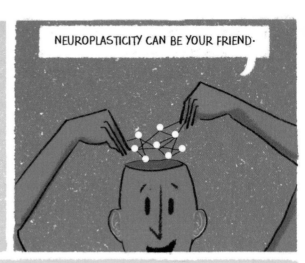

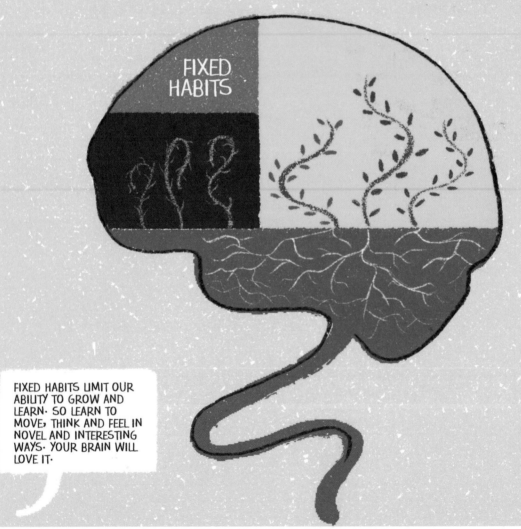

'Stereotyping is the enemy - exercise the brain with a variety of movement, action and challenge' (Merzenich 2013).

Michael Merzenich is a huge figure in the science of neuroplasticity. He is very optimistic about our ability to enhance the functioning of our 'soft wired' nervous system.

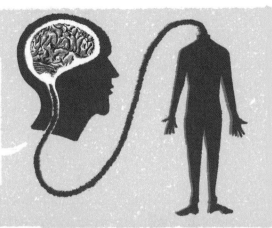

BRAINS NEED TO BE REMINDED OF THE REAL BODY ALL THE TIME. THE BODY NEUROTAG NEEDS CONSTANT FEEDING OR OUR 'VIRTUAL BODY' BECOMES MORE ABSTRACT.

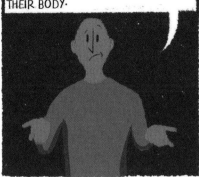

ONE OF THE BIGGEST INSIGHTS I HAVE HAD FROM CLINICAL EXPERIENCE IS MOST PEOPLE ARE POOR AT FEELING THEIR BODY.

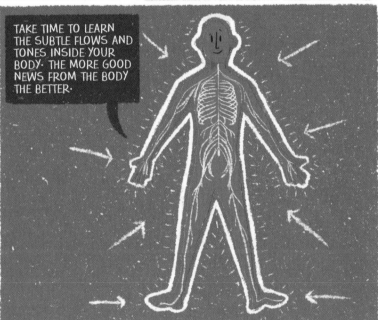

TAKE TIME TO LEARN THE SUBTLE FLOWS AND TONES INSIDE YOUR BODY. THE MORE GOOD NEWS FROM THE BODY THE BETTER.

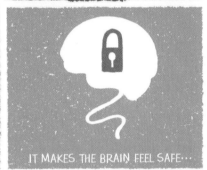

IT MAKES THE BRAIN FEEL SAFE...

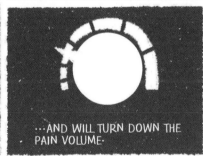

...AND WILL TURN DOWN THE PAIN VOLUME.

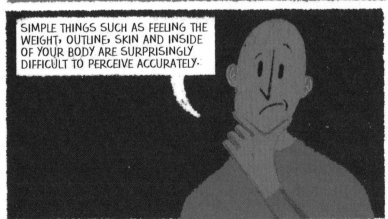

SIMPLE THINGS SUCH AS FEELING THE WEIGHT, OUTLINE, SKIN AND INSIDE OF YOUR BODY ARE SURPRISINGLY DIFFICULT TO PERCEIVE ACCURATELY.

IT IS USEFUL TO REDUCE THE SENSATION YOU EXPERIENCE TO REALLY SIMPLE DESCRIPTIVE WORDS. IS IT HOT OR COLD, MOVING OR FIXED, QUICK OR SLOW, BIG OR SMALL? PAIN MAY BECOME A 'WARM, PULSING AREA THE SIZE OF A PLUM'.

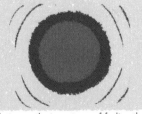

'We don't need a body to feel a body.' This is the amazing conclusion of pain pioneer Ronald Melzack (Melzack and Katz 2013). Treatments that use skillful touch can really help you find your body.

There is lots of evidence accumulating on the importance of feeling the slow background tone of your body (interoception) as well as joints and muscles (proprioception). It takes practice to sense your organs and the internal feel of your limbs, but doing so will pay you back in dividends.

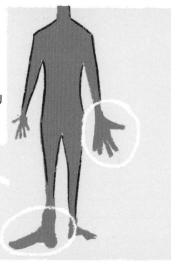

THE SUBJECTIVE SENSE OF THE BODY CAN BE CALLED A BODY MAP.

BODY MAPS ARE FREQUENTLY DISTORTED WHEN YOU ASK OR TEST PEOPLE ON THEIR PERCEPTION OF THE BODY.

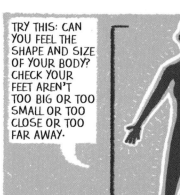

TRY THIS: CAN YOU FEEL THE SHAPE AND SIZE OF YOUR BODY? CHECK YOUR FEET AREN'T TOO BIG OR TOO SMALL OR TOO CLOSE OR TOO FAR AWAY.

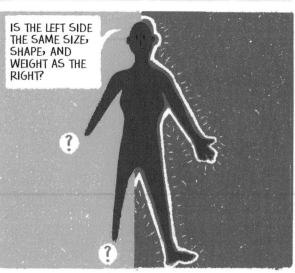

IS THE LEFT SIDE THE SAME SIZE, SHAPE, AND WEIGHT AS THE RIGHT?

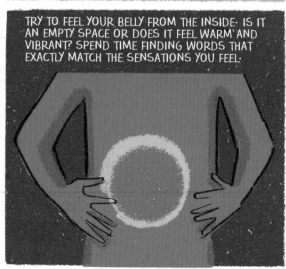

TRY TO FEEL YOUR BELLY FROM THE INSIDE. IS IT AN EMPTY SPACE OR DOES IT FEEL WARM AND VIBRANT? SPEND TIME FINDING WORDS THAT EXACTLY MATCH THE SENSATIONS YOU FEEL.

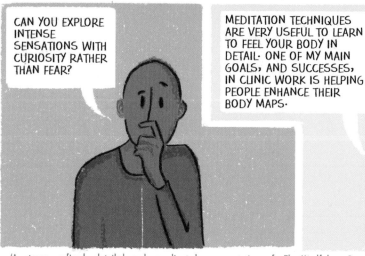

CAN YOU EXPLORE INTENSE SENSATIONS WITH CURIOSITY RATHER THAN FEAR?

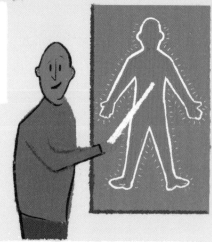

MEDITATION TECHNIQUES ARE VERY USEFUL TO LEARN TO FEEL YOUR BODY IN DETAIL. ONE OF MY MAIN GOALS, AND SUCCESSES, IN CLINIC WORK IS HELPING PEOPLE ENHANCE THEIR BODY MAPS.

'A strong, refined, detailed and coordinated representation of information from any given region of your body is, by its fundamental nature, anti-pain' (Merzenich 2013).

The Mindfulness-Based Stress Reduction model is an accessible, researched, and secular meditation method (Kabat-Zinn 2013). Zen Mind Beginner's Mind (Suzuki 1970) is an enduring classic on doing less and achieving more.

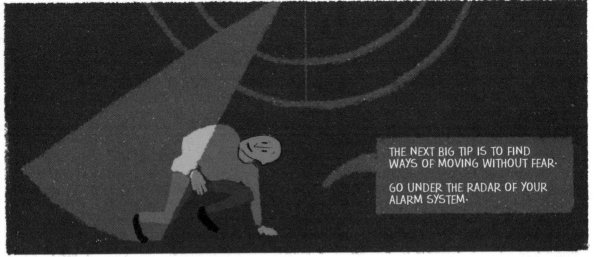

THE NEXT BIG TIP IS TO FIND WAYS OF MOVING WITHOUT FEAR.

GO UNDER THE RADAR OF YOUR ALARM SYSTEM.

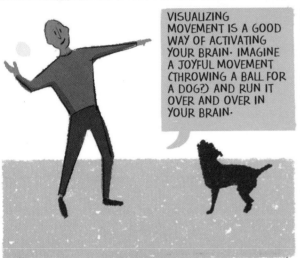

VISUALIZING MOVEMENT IS A GOOD WAY OF ACTIVATING YOUR BRAIN. IMAGINE A JOYFUL MOVEMENT (THROWING A BALL FOR A DOG?) AND RUN IT OVER AND OVER IN YOUR BRAIN.

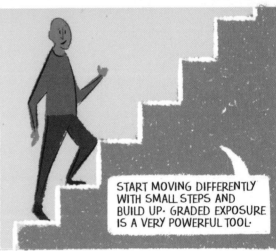

START MOVING DIFFERENTLY WITH SMALL STEPS AND BUILD UP. GRADED EXPOSURE IS A VERY POWERFUL TOOL.

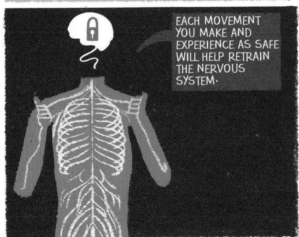

EACH MOVEMENT YOU MAKE AND EXPERIENCE AS SAFE WILL HELP RETRAIN THE NERVOUS SYSTEM.

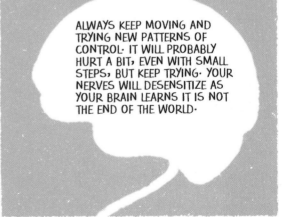

ALWAYS KEEP MOVING AND TRYING NEW PATTERNS OF CONTROL. IT WILL PROBABLY HURT A BIT, EVEN WITH SMALL STEPS, BUT KEEP TRYING. YOUR NERVES WILL DESENSITIZE AS YOUR BRAIN LEARNS IT IS NOT THE END OF THE WORLD.

'The feelings and the thoughts about movement are inseparable from the movement itself' (Merzenich 2012). 'Graded exposure often involves using creativity to find alternative ways to painlessly perform a movement that is normally painful.' 'It gives the brain good news' (Hargrove 2014).

'We don't know which exercise programmes are best, but almost everything we try is getting them moving. It is important that the programmes contain education to reconceptualise pain as protective, and that the participants have a strong message that they are not broken' (Rovner 2014, World Congress on Pain).

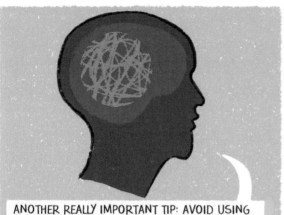

ANOTHER REALLY IMPORTANT TIP: AVOID USING LANGUAGE THAT MESSES WITH YOUR BRAIN. YOU CAN CHANGE THE PAIN NEUROTAG WITH NEW LANGUAGE AND CONCEPTS.

EXPLORE HOW YOU UNDERSTAND WHY YOU ARE IN PAIN. 'MY MUSCLES ARE REALLY TIGHT.' SO THEN, WHAT IS THE EXACT OPPOSITE OF TIGHT FOR YOU?

AN EXAMPLE OF UNHELPFUL LANGUAGE IS 'SLIPPED DISCS'. THEY SOUND SCARY, BUT THEY CAN NEVER HAPPEN. MAYBE USE THE METAPHOR OF A DISC UNDER PRESSURE OR SOMETHING BEING SQUEEZED, AND THEN FOCUS ON REDUCING THE PRESSURE AND HOW TO UNSQUEEZE.

MUCH LESS SCARY.

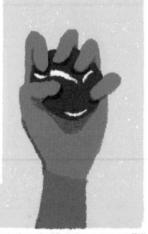

ANYTHING THAT DE-THREATENS THE SENSATIONS YOU ARE FEELING AND SUPPORTS NEW POSSIBILITIES WILL HELP BREAK THE PAIN HABIT. SELL YOURSELF MORE BEAUTIFUL, ELEGANT AND ACCURATE STORIES.

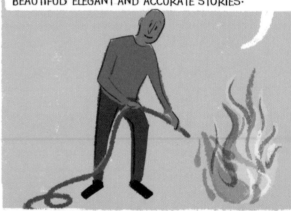

PLAY WITH METAPHORS THAT FIT YOU BUT OFFER THE POSSIBILITY OF CHANGE. AVOID PAIN AS AN EXTERNAL THING, PAIN AS VIOLENCE AND DAMAGE, PAIN AS YOUR FAULT (YOU DO NOT DESERVE TO SUFFER!) OR PAIN AS A BATTLE. THESE METAPHORS RARELY HELP.

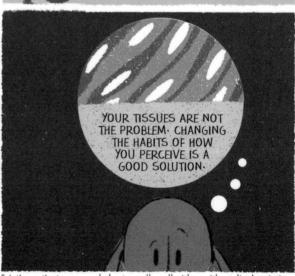

YOUR TISSUES ARE NOT THE PROBLEM. CHANGING THE HABITS OF HOW YOU PERCEIVE IS A GOOD SOLUTION.

If you've ever seen a disc in a cadaver you can't slip the suckers, they're immobile, but that's our language and it messes with your brain' (Moseley 2014).

Sciatica patients recovered about equally well with or without disc herniations visible on MRI scans in a large study in the New England Journal of Medicine (el Barzouhi et al 2013).

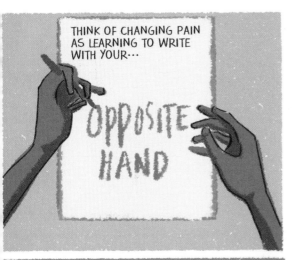

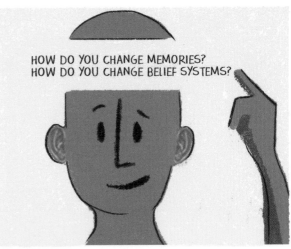

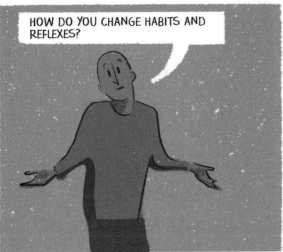

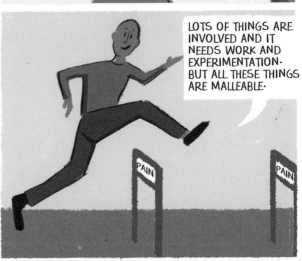

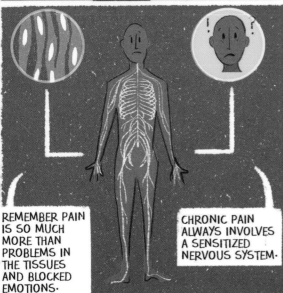

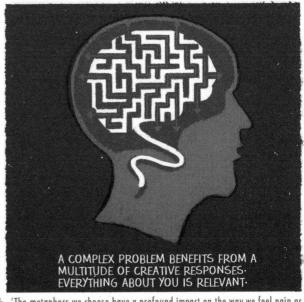

For leading pain theorist David Butler, co-author of the hugely influential book Explain Pain, changing metaphors is a central tool in changing the pain experience (Butler 2013).

'The metaphors we choose have a profound impact on the way we feel pain as well as upon the ways our suffering is treated' (Bourke 2014).

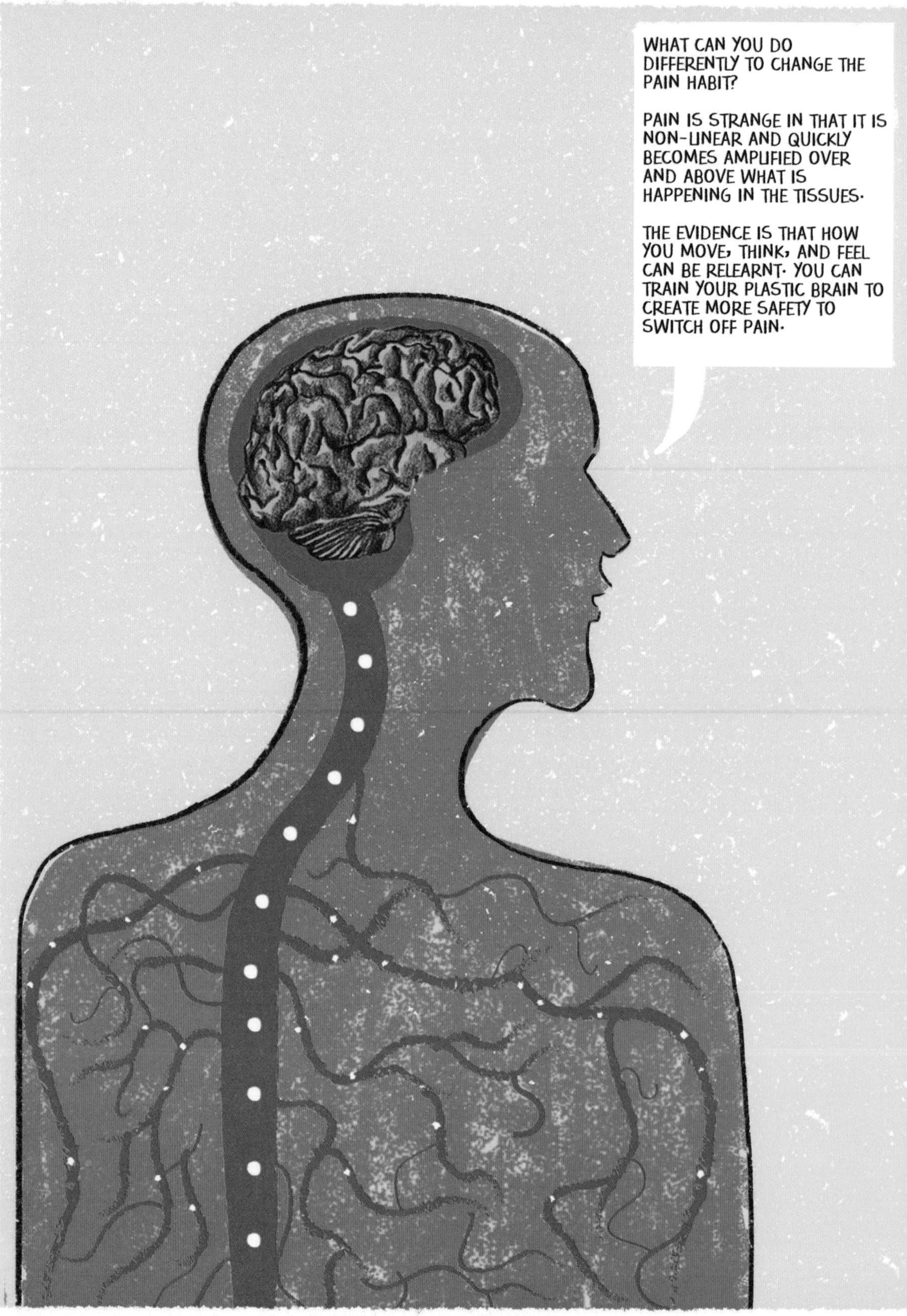
WHAT CAN YOU DO DIFFERENTLY TO CHANGE THE PAIN HABIT?
PAIN IS STRANGE IN THAT IT IS NON-LINEAR AND QUICKLY BECOMES AMPLIFIED OVER AND ABOVE WHAT IS HAPPENING IN THE TISSUES.
THE EVIDENCE IS THAT HOW YOU MOVE, THINK, AND FEEL CAN BE RELEARNT. YOU CAN TRAIN YOUR PLASTIC BRAIN TO CREATE MORE SAFETY TO SWITCH OFF PAIN.

REFERENCES

Bourke J (2014a) The Story of Pain: From Prayer to Painkillers. Oxford University Press.

Bourke J (2014b) BBC Radio Interview. www.bbc.co.uk/programmes/b046j8z5, accessed 2015-02-10

Brainman (2014) Understanding Pain: Brainman Stops His Opioids. youtube.com, http://bit.ly/brainman-opioids, accessed 2015-02-10

Butler DS (2013) The Linguistic Journey and Pain. noijam.com, http://bit.ly/2c2sFEo, accessed 2015-02-10

Butler DS, and Moseley GL (2003) Explain Pain. www.noigroup.com, accessed 2015-02-10

Cervero F (2012) Understanding Pain: Exploring the Perception of Pain. MIT Press.

Dunn WR et al (2014) Symptoms of Pain Do Not Correlate with Rotator Cuff Tear Severity. J Bone Joint Surg Am, 96(10): 793–800.

el Barzouhi A et al (2013) Magnetic Resonance Imaging in Follow-up Assessment of Sciatica. N Engl J Med, 368: 999–1007.

Hargrove T (2014) A Guide to Better Movement. www.bettermovement.org

Huffington Post (2012) Manteo Mitchell Broken Leg: U.S. 4x400M Runner Finishes Olympic Relay after Breaking Leg. Huffington Post, Eddie Pells. http://bit.ly/huffpo-mitchell-broke-leg, accessed 2015-02-10

Ingraham P (2011) Pain Changes How Pain Works. www.painscience.com, http://bit.ly/2bwW1W8, accessed 2015-02-10

Ingraham P (2014) Your Back Is Not Out of Alignment. www.painscience.com, http://bit.ly/2bM3T8c, accessed 2015-02-09

Kabat-Zinn J (2013) Full Catastrophe Living, Revised Edition. Piatkus.

Kirton A et al (2008). Seizure Response Dogs: Evaluation of a Formal Training Program. Epilepsy Behav, 13(3): 499–504.

Krane E (2011) The Mystery of Chronic Pain. www.TED.com, accessed 2014-10-14

Lederman E (2010) The Fall of the Postural–Structural–Biomechanical Model in Manual and Physical Therapies: Exemplified by Lower Back Pain. CPDO Online Journal, 1–14.

Levine P, and Phillips M (2012) Freedom from Pain. Discover Your Body's Power to Overcome Physical Pain. Sounds True.

Louw A (2013) Why Do I Hurt? www.ispinstitute.com, accessed 2015-02-10

Louw A (2014) Teaching People About Pain. Institute for Chronic Pain. http://bit.ly/louw-descartes-wrong, accessed 2015-02-10

Medical News Today (2014) Dogs 'Sniff Out Prostate Cancer with 98% Accuracy', Study Finds. http://bit.ly/2beZ9Kv, accessed 2015-02-10

Melzack R, and Katz J (2013) Pain. WIREs Cogn Sci, 4: 1–15.

Merzenich M (2012) Dr. Michael Merzenich on Neuroscience, Learning and the Feldenkrais Method. www.bettermovement.org, http://bit.ly/2bssAY6, accessed 2013-05-01

Merzenich M (2013) Soft-Wired. Parnassus Publishing.

Michaleff et al (2014) Comprehensive Physiotherapy Exercise Programme or Advice for Chronic Whiplash. The Lancet, 384(9938): 133–141.

Moseley GL (2003) A Pain Neuromatrix Approach to Patients with Chronic Pain. Manual Therapy. 8(3): 130–140.

Moseley GL (2012a) Teaching People about Pain: Why Do We Keep Beating Around the Bush? Pain Management, 2(1): 1–3.

Moseley GL (2012b) Pain Really Is in the Mind, But Not in the Way You Think. www.theconversation.com, http://bit.ly/1neyk45, accessed 2015-02-10

Moseley GL (2014) You Can't Slip a Disc, Spinal Herniation Probably Doesn't Really Matter, and Your Alignment Doesn't Mean as Much as You Think. Blood and Iron Blog. http://bit.ly/cant-slip-a-disc, accessed 2015-02-10

Rovner G (2014) World Congress on Pain Comes to You. 6: Physical Activity and Chronic Pain. www.bodyinmind.org/physical-activity-chronic-pain, accessed 2014-12-10

Sandkühler J, and Lee J (2013) How to Erase Memory Traces of Pain and Fear. Trends in Neuroscience, 36(6): 343–352.

Suzuki S (1970) Zen Mind, Beginner's Mind. Weatherhill.

Thacker MA et al (2007) Pathophysiology of Peripheral Neuropathic Pain: Immune Cells and Molecules. IARS, 105(3).

Wall P (2000) Pain: The Science of Suffering. Columbia University Press.

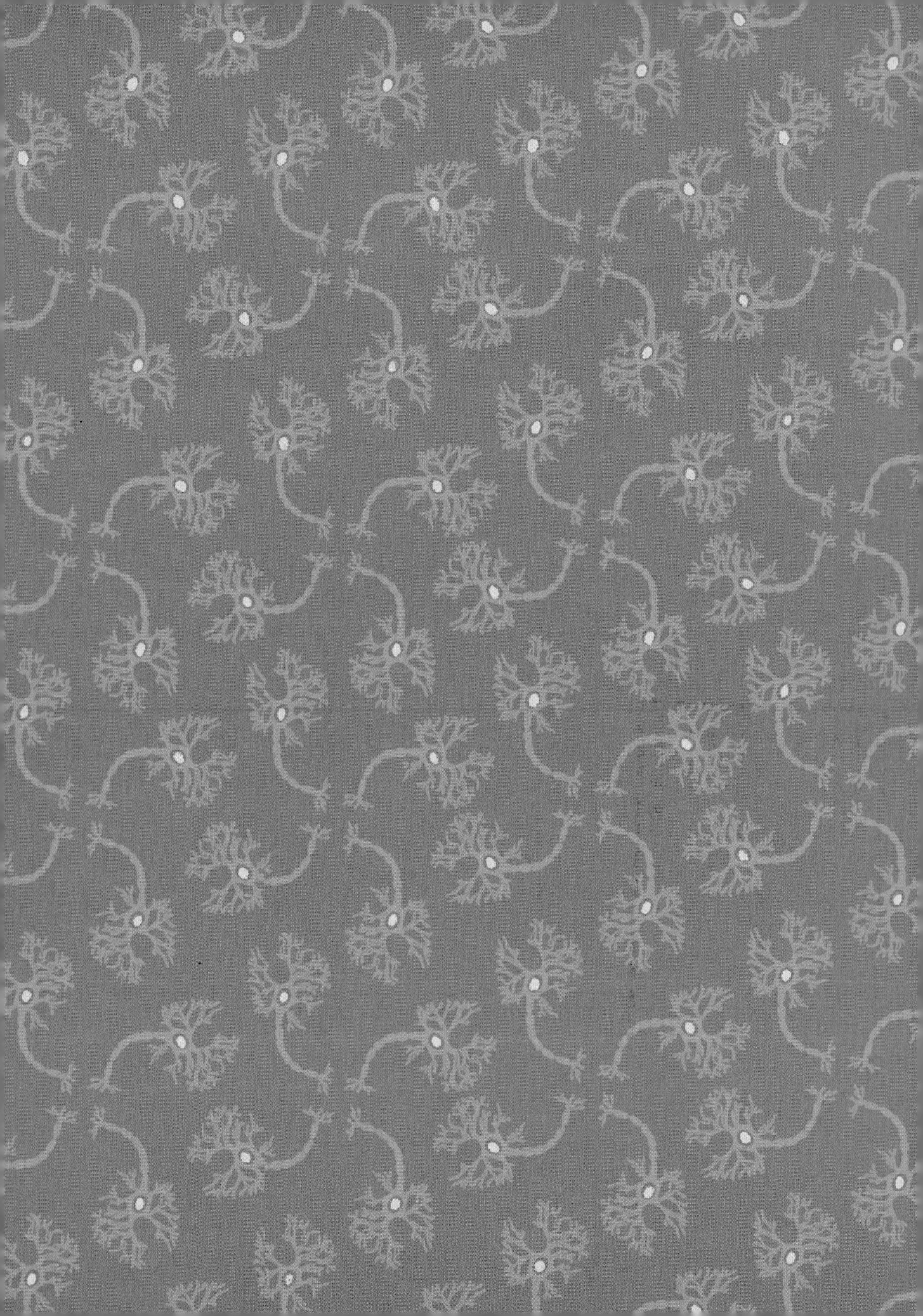